THE HEALING HANDS OF REIKI

AN INTRODUCTION TO REIKI

ANGELA GLASER

Made with ♥ on the Notion Press Platform
www.notionpress.com

Contents

1. Introduction   1

2. The Origin Of Reiki   3

3. The Ideals Of Reiki – Exploring The Principles   6

4. How Does Reiki Help? – Taking Charge Of Your Health   10

5. The Art Of Mastering The Therapy   15

6. Final Take On The Energy Healing   20

Disclaimer   23

1

Introduction

What is Reiki? Try and ask this question to anyone who has ever heard about Reiki. Odds are, you will get an answer that it is a therapy used to heal an existing condition that is out of balance.

In last couple of years this art of healing has gained a huge popularity amongst lot of people worldwide. The recipients, who have experienced this natural healing art first-hand, have described how it expresses the energy to the receiver to help restore stability, thereby helping in healing emotional and physical stress. In other words, Reiki is a way to promote relaxation and ease the level of stress in human body.

Reiki was originally discovered in Japan, but over the years it has become quite popular in the western countries and other parts of the world. Reiki is often termed as a "gift of the creator" - a caring gift that has the ability of altering your life and the lives of your loved ones. However, Reiki is more powerful than the healing art. In the last decade thousands of people have been touched by this healing therapy and the irony is, many would not even be aware of the significant changes that have been bought to their lives by a Reiki professional.

One of the most important benefits of Reiki is its power to direct your life in a direction that is correct for you. Try using Reiki in your difficult situations. You would realise that the guidance of what you do, comes very easily. Most importantly, it changes your attitude towards a particular situation. All of a sudden, you would see a complete new perspective of your condition.

So, Reiki is nothing but a healing therapy that provides you energy to overcome your problems. There are some misconceptions about the therapy about what it is and what is not. Let us begin our journey to this wonderful, yet least explained, power of energy.

2
The Origin of Reiki

Unlike other therapies that involves ingestion or application of artificial substances in human body, Reiki is more spiritual and vibration healing practice that maintains balance throughout human body. That is the reason it is known as the hand-healing practice.

Everyone has their own reasons to receive or practice Reiki. Some take it to strengthen their health, while some receive it to fight the negative forces in the body or in order to support their medical care. People who receive Reiki often express a sense of correlation to their own inherent spirituality. However, Reiki is not a religion. There are no religious belief systems attached to Reiki.

So, how it all started?

Where does it come from?

Reiki is typically a sort of hands on healing, with its genesis in India plus the East dating back a lot of thousands of years to the time ahead of Christ and Buddha.

Reiki is practiced across all parts of the globe today, however the teaching dates back to early 1920's in Japan. Mikao Usui is the man who discovered the root system called Reiki. Today, his teachings and practices are passed through several Reiki grandmasters.

Usui was a spiritual man, a monk with a wife and two children. During his era, practices of Buddhists and Shinto were quite prevalent in Japan's tradition and culture. It was 1922, when Usui decided to exercise his intense spiritual practices that concluded into a philosophical revelation called Reiki today. He was quite determined to learn the secret healing so that it helps in curing others and which took him on a journey to several countries.

During his journey, he travelled to the mountains of Kori Yama, a sacred mountain outside Koyoto, where he fasted for almost 21 days in order to achieve a high changed state of awareness which he thought would allow him with the curing power. However by the 21st day, Dr Usui started getting frustrated and decided to discontinue the meditation, when a sudden spiritual energy ran down from top of his head to the bottom, thereby making him enlightened.

Dr Usui learnt and practiced healing of the spirit; however, it was during his learning he realised that his learning's are more focussed on healing of the body and not the spirit. Hence he truly believed; people who could hold close a life of complete healing could only benefit from Reiki. Therefore, he decided to treat only those people who are ready to commit towards mental and physical healing.

Later Dr Chujiro Hayashi continued his practices by opening a Reiki clinic. During his tenure, he developed new techniques of Reiki which had the same impressions of energy and lineage as Dr Usui Reiki. Today Reiki is taught with more proper phases which include hand positions and science based practices within Reiki.

Thought behind the Therapy

Since Reiki was discovered by a Japanese founder, Dr Mikao Usui, therefore you could find deep impressions of Japanese techniques in the therapy.

As mentioned earlier, Reiki is a technique to reduce stress and provide relaxation to mind, body and soul that promotes healing. The process of healing is administered by "positioning of hands" and is based on the idea that an invisible power of energy flows through our body that keeps us alive. The word Reiki is derived from two Japanese words, where Rei means "Universal" and Ki means "life force energy". So, it won't be wrong to say Reiki as religiously channelled life force energy.

The best way to know about Reiki is to talk to the people who have undergone the miraculous treatment themselves. These recipients have expressed a feeling of happiness that flows within and around them. It does not solely works on the body but it also benefits emotions, mind and spirits thereby relaxing the mood and enhancing the feeling of peace and good health.

Unlike other treatments, Reiki is simple and natural method of spiritual curing. It has been successful in serving practically every known disease and problem and constantly creates a positive outcome. Moreover, it works in combination amid all other therapeutic procedures to alleviate side-effects and encourage healing.

3

The Ideals of Reiki — Exploring the principles

The ideologies of Reiki are essential for the practice and understanding of the healing therapy. One should not forget that Reiki was and still is a strong tool, not just for healing purposes but also for spiritual and personal growth of the human being. Although Reiki does not follow any religion, it could be practiced by people of any faith and in order to get most out of your experience, whether it is it by giving to someone or receiving from someone, you should aspire to live by the principles of Reiki. After all, it is a life choice.

The world of Reiki is based on five fundamental principles of Reiki, which was originally established on the philosophies of Meiji King of Japan during the 18th century and later, was adopted by the founding father of Reiki, Dr Mikao Usui. Currently, there are hundreds of schools that teach Reiki and each has its own techniques of practicing. However, they all are derived from the initial teachings of Mikao Usui and have their own versions with similar meanings at their core:

- *"Just for today, do not anger"*
- *"Just for today, do not worry."*

- *"Just for today, honour you parents, teachers and elders"*
- *"Just for today, earn your living honestly"*
- *"Just for today, show gratitude to every living thing"*

Just for today, do not anger:

Every day is different. There are times when we all are unhappy about something and this principle is all about knowing the ways to transform the anger. As human beings, we often try to suppress our anger that can be destructive and more powerful than before. In our fit of anger, we often try to hide our emotions, such as fear. So, it is important to understand the reason of our anger and realise what does it actually mean as this can be the first steps towards transforming your anger in a positive direction. As human beings, we have little or no control over our anger and it takes lot of patience and determination to change the habitual harmful response into a composed and conscious positive action.

Just for today, do not worry:

Why do we worry? May be because we do not trust or may be because we presume that the things would not shape in the manner we thought or planned. But the truth is, most of the things that worry us do NOT happen! And even if they do, worrying would not help.

This is not surprising. Right from our childhood we are conditioned in a way that we should compete with each other and we start making efforts to make things work as per us. This feeling cultivates a lack of trust in the world around us. Bizarrely enough, the act of distressing drains the very energy out of our body which we might need to deal with circumstances like trauma or catastrophe. So, you need to take suitable actions to reduce the stress of worry and try to work out on the principle that at least for one day, we would let all our worries go. Worry is nothing but a fear of consequences of past events or fear of the future, how things might turn in future that may hurt us. So, don't hold the past and trust in god to provide for the future. Live in the present. That is the reason it says, "Just for today"

Just for today, honour your parents, teachers and elders:

I believe, this is the first lesson that is taught in our childhood days as part of morality - be kind and respect others.

Compassion and respect for us and others is the first step to the journey of spirituality. As kids, we are raised to look up to our elders and listen and respect our teachers and parents. However, as we grow we often forget this simple rule of humbleness. So, "just for today", try to listen and respect other, it might surprise you.

Just for today, earn your living honestly:

We all know that the world is a crooked place and we all need to be smart enough to deal with muggers around us. It sometimes gets difficult to work honestly and earn our living. This is because we have that lack of trust in our abilities and the abilities of the people around us.

Once a sage was asked, is it possible to know how prosperous a person could be? He thought deeply and then replied, the amount of prosperity in an individual can be measured by the fact that how much or in what quantity of peace does a person carry in their heart. In order to earn our livings honestly, we need to honest in our dealings. People who believe in earning honestly, they are not only honest to themselves but also to the world around them. They have that trust in their own capabilities to earn the amount of living they need for them and their families. These kinds of people have more peace in their heart and are more prosperous in life.

While creating this principle, Dr Usui believed that honesty is a heavy burden to carry and if a person wants to live peacefully and happily, they must have the ability to align themselves fully with their life's purpose.

Just for today, show gratitude to every living thing:

Have you ever thought, do we really thank other people for helping us? Not really! In today's world we all are in a race to get the best of our lives and this race encourages us to want more and more. We often forget to thank even ourselves for what we actually have. It takes lot of patience and perseverance to move from "Can I have" to "thank god for what I have". This kind of transformation is a real revelation.

Being humble and grateful is important to lead a happy life. Life is a blessing, so just for today, be grateful to it, acknowledge it and say thanks for it.

Therefore, the mantra to live a happy life is to live in the Reiki principals, which teach us "just for today"....which means, today is now. Live sensibly now, yesterday is history and future is yet to come. The ideologies of Dr Usui tell us to live in the present and don't look back in the past and cry or wishing for an opportunity that isn't there yet. Be grateful of what you have today and live life celebrating in the magnificence of today.

4

How does Reiki Help? – Taking charge of your Health

By now we are aware of the fact that Reiki is an energy healing treatment that works on complete mind, body and soul. Reiki is not a religion and does not work under any systems of religious beliefs. It is a way to relax your mind with the help of natural healing vibrations that are transmitted from the hands of the Reiki practitioner to the body of the receiver.

Let us understand how Reiki actually helps in uplifting our emotions and wellbeing.

How does it work?

We all know that happiness has a direct relation with our health. A healthy person is able to survive certain amount of stress and then bounces back. This happens because our body has internal healing abilities that include various self-regulating methods to maintain the overall balance.

However, if we receive constant sudden or intense stress over a period of time, our body's self-regulating mechanism starts failing. In other words, our body's ability to normalize itself becomes compromised, thereby resulting in declining of our health. There is only so much that our body can take. This constant bearing of stress causes our body to lose its capacity to rebalance. Unless taken seriously, the stresses of everyday life – be it physical, mental or social, can merge with an individual's tendency to fight and can result in health deteriorating.

This is the time when this simple and natural process of healing through Reiki helps. The treatment helps in reducing the impact of stress on the body and release tension from the entire system. Once the recipient receives the treatment, not only he/she move upwards towards his/her own unique balance of mind, body and soul, but also, it starts recuperating body's self-regulating mechanisms. The body's own healing processes begin to function more effectively.

What does Reiki do?

Reiki is channelling the energy from the healer to the healee, a treatment, a way of leading a healthy life.

As energy, it helps in maintaining the strength of the mind and universal life force. When we hand over ourselves into the hand of a reiki practitioner, we allow our body to balance subtle energies. The more the energy is balanced, the more our life is balanced. It helps our body to nurse back to health from within. So, it won't be wrong to say that Reiki is an intelligent energy and knows exactly where it is most needed. Possibilities are, we might not want be where we want it to go, but wherever it goes, it is always for the maximum good. The recipient who has experienced this healing energy has expressed, Reiki is a current or a vibration felt in the body. It can feel like a breeze or a wave. There may be times when we might not feel it, but is always working on us.

As a therapy, it helps in relieving stress and discharges any kind of energy disorders in our body. If our body experience any kind of energy disruptions, we feel emotional and physical symptoms like:

- Nervousness
- Allergy-like reactions, asthma, and eczema
- Unbearable pain
- Disquiet
- Stress and anxiety
- Stomach ache
- Dejection
- Addictive behaviour
- Panic attacks or unnecessary worry
- Cancer, heart attacks, and stroke
- Anger and unease
- Extreme remorse and embarrassment

During the Reiki treatment, the Reiki master places his/her hand on you or in the air above your body. He/she then channels the Reiki energy from them to you. In this process, the energy is channelled through the healer and not from the healer. The practitioner acts as conduit for the energy.

What it feels like?

As Reiki energies flow between the healer and the healee, therefore both the bodies can react or respond to the sensations. Usually these sensations are pleasant. You could feel different kinds of emotions flowing through your body like warm, cold, faithfulness or forcefulness. So, you could actually feel the energies flowing, it does not matter whether you are giving it or receiving it. This feeling acts like a verification that the energy is welcomed in your body.

Reiki treatment works like a thermostat that regulates the body temperature. The Reiki energy can flow rapidly or slowly as needed to distribute balancing energies. These fluctuations in the body can often be felt like insects moving or pins and needles tingling, goose bumps or hot flashes. During the treatment, both the practitioner and the recipient must work like a team. They should feel the Reiki sensations. Possibilities are, because the energies flow through the hands of the practitioner, it might warm up his/her hands - an indication that energy is flowing seamlessly. During the course of the treatment, the recipient might feel sleepy; this is because it helps in draining the stress out of the body, thus calming the internal energies.

Reiki would work best on the people are ready to commit mentally and physically to the healer. A person needs to relax during the treatment. However, sometimes there could be some healing reactions like, discomfort or tears. If you get this tearful feeling, let it happen, it would soon pass. Tears are kind of energy disruptions that are released from the body during the treatment. Some people even laugh or giggle during the treatment. DON'T be embarrassed. It is OK to have this feeling. There would be times when you don't feel anything at all. That is OK too. For Reiki to work, it does not require you to feel anything. It often works in a subtle manner. It is not like taking a tablet for a pain and feeling the results in thirty minutes. However, once you are through with the treatment, it might feel as if it was the right thing to do in that moment of time.

So how the treatment of Reiki does actually helps in healing stress and tension from the body? This is one question that is yet to be answered. However, there is ample amount of documentation to prove the effects of Reiki such as lowering blood pressure or reduce rate of heart attacks.

For any treatment to work, the receiver should trust in the treatment and believe that the treatment would help. Don't forget to attend the number of sessions as guided by your specialist. It is similar to taking the full course of medicine. If you break the course in between, the medicine would not cure you completely. Similarly, unless you take the complete sessions, the Reiki might not be as helpful as it should be. Also, since there are no side-effects of Reiki, it makes it suitable for everyone of any age and at any time.

Reiki as a way of life is exact explanation that potentially boosts you up to the point of pure joy. If you plan to learn Reiki, a good Reiki practitioner would teach the techniques to carry out the discipline of self-healing and meditation. They would also teach you the ways to incorporate the five ideologies of Reiki into your life. By incorporating Reiki principles in your life and living according to them, you can feel yourself in a position of calmness and elevating the mood that is truly amazing. This brings us to our next section of how can you practice Reiki.

5
The Art of Mastering the Therapy

Being a system of curing and spiritual growth, Reiki has enjoyed considerable recognition and success globally. Originated in Japan, almost a century ago, this practice has now been taught to millions across the world.

The fundamentals of Reiki can be transmitted between nine to eleven hours, which is the greatest advantage of Reiki. People who have attended the sessions are easily able to deliver the therapy to themselves and their loved ones after a weekend class or short evening sessions. Since there are no side effects, hence it is as safe as giving massage to someone and they can do this responsibly.

Your Reiki Connection

There could be hundreds of reasons; why you might be considering Reiki. May be because a friend suggested you or may be because you have seen effects of Reiki on your neighbour post the therapy. There could also be a reason that you have always been attached to spirituality and energies flowing within and around you or perhaps because you may be sensitive to the medications you have been using to treat your illness and now looking for something subtler to treat you.

There are countless reasons why people turn towards the treatment of Reiki and some might be just simply drawn towards it. Whatever might be the reason, it has helped you deciding whether to receive the treatment or if you would want to pioneer yourself in this practice.

How to Incorporate Reiki in your life?

There are two ways through which you can bring the art of healing in your life – either by receiving the treatment or by giving the treatment to someone as a Reiki Master. One of the biggest strength of this therapy is that you need not to have specific degrees or education to pursue it. You can learn Reiki yourself so that anytime when you feel that you need a treatment, you can give it yourself. Many Reiki professionals even encourage their students or patients to practice and learn Reiki for self care, especially to those who are suffering from serious illness or lead a very stressful life.

One of the most wonderful things about Reiki is that it only helps. There are no counter effects of this therapy. You cannot complain about a Reiki overdose, no matter how many treatments or sessions you have gone through.

Why do you need to learn Reiki?

It is more relaxing to receive a massage from someone rather than giving it (though some people find it relaxing by giving massage), similarly, Reiki is a wonderful experience when received from someone else. Usually self-care is valued more by people who have health challenges; however, it can also be beneficial for people who lead a stressful life and are seeking more balance in their life.

Learning self-care Reiki can help those with chronic diseases like asthma, diabetes, epilepsy, depression, heart disease etc. They can even practice Reiki on themselves in order to release tension and reduce stress, as well as, enhancing their own health.

How can you learn Self-Car Reiki?

The best way to learn Reiki for self-care or for the treatments of your near and dear ones is through a Reiki master.

One of the easiest ways to find the right trainer for yourself is to ask your friends who have been practicing this therapy. Another way could be talking to practitioners of the same genre like acupuncture or Shaistu. Normally these people would know about the other complementary therapy providers. But before finalizing your own Reiki expert, you need to understand that it is not a standardized practice and hence does not guarantee that someone who is claiming to be the Reiki Master is actually have relevant experience in teaching Reiki. Therefore, it is important to check the background and the credibility of the teacher before finalizing it.

At the end, you should confirm from the Reiki master for opportunities they would offer for continued practice and mentoring. So choose the Reiki master carefully. Do not just simply go by the experience but also look for someone with whom you can build a rapport.

Becoming a Reiki Master yourself

Apart from using Reiki on yourself, you can become a master yourself. All it requires is that determination and commitment towards the training and techniques involved in the training.

In order to become a Reiki expert yourself, you need to undergo three levels of practice. Nevertheless, the key to become an expert yourself lies in the daily hands on practice of self treatment at all levels of practice.

- **First Degree Reiki Training:Speciality – Self-care**

In this level, students who want to learn Reiki would require to learn self-care with each other. In this session, students learn to incorporate Reiki in their daily life by using the techniques themselves. Other than self-care training, they also learn to use hands positions when treating their family members. This can be achieved either by one full session or shortened chair session. Apart from this, they are also taught to use Reiki in extreme situations. In case you are a medical professional or a nurse, your Reiki sessions would take place in a proper clinical setting, where you would be taught to apply Reiki with medical terms.

The ultimate goal of the Reiki Master is to encourage students to become the channel for passing the Reiki energy. People who do not want to pursue it professionally and want to be limited to self-care or treating family or friends to the utmost, first degree Reiki training is all they need.

- **Second Degree Reiki Training: Speciality – Distant Healing**

This is the more advanced way of becoming a Reiki professional because it requires students to learn to substitute the hand to body contact through a psychological bond when needed so that healing can be accessible when it is impossible to touch the recipient. That is why it is known as distant healing. However, the second degree training is not only limited to distant healing. Its techniques and methods can be used for hand-on practice.

- **Third Degree Reiki Training:Speciality – becoming the Reiki Master**

This is the third and the last level of mastering the art of healing, becoming a Reiki Master. In earlier days, this level of training was only done via invitation only. The reason to this was, the aim was to teach people who are ready to commit their lives in teaching people to practice Reiki. The traditional learning of Reiki in this degree does not happen through course work; rather it happens through an extended studentship with a Reiki master. Only post completing all the three level of training, one can become a Reiki master who can pass on their teachings to others.

Hence, it does not matter whether you learn Reiki to treat yourself or others, all it requires is some commitment and devotion to this practice. Learning Reiki is not difficult and does not involve of reading books and clearing exams. In order to be proficient with Reiki, you need to self-practice at all levels. Do not just jump levels as it would not lead to your goal of healing.

6
Final take on the Energy Healing

Finally what I think is, Reiki is a treatment that is wonderful to receive as well as to give. The first lesson that it teaches us is understand the value of trust. It is best to let the energy flow on its own rather than suppressing it or controlling it. Remember we spoke about Reiki being an intelligent therapy! It knows where to go and what to do.

People who are sensitive to the treatment often complain that, when they focus too hard on the techniques or try to control Reiki, in all possibilities they are restricting the flow of energy. So you need to keep aside all the controls and start trusting on the energy and let it do what it needs to do, let it go where it needs to go in order to achieve increased sense of well-being and increase the benefits of the treatment.

The second lesson what Reiki has taught us today is the importance of invoking control, showing gratitude to others, working honestly and not to worry unless required and the ways to calm your senses. So it arises another question, do you really need to believe in Reiki?

The answer is NO. You need not to believe in anything for it to work. All it required you to be open-minded in order to experience the magic of healing energy. Reiki is not a religion. It does not require you to adhere to any particular set of beliefs. Reiki is a life choice and comes with no rules. Reiki means energy of life. Everything in the world including plants and animals has Reiki in them. Perhaps the actual definition of Reiki is yet to be answered because it is not easy to define something which is invisible yet very powerful. Using Reiki is all about harnessing t the energy that dwells within us.

In this book, we have used the word treatment many times; however, we do not want you to think that Reiki should be seen as a substitute to the traditional medicine. The practice of Reiki works by encouraging harmony and balance in the body and a Reiki professional would never diagnose to offer treatment for a specific disorder. Rather it helps in healing the body itself.

The biggest strength of Reiki is that it can be practiced by anyone and can pursue the levels as per their requirements. It does not require any special skills or even to be a religious person. All you need to build is the connection to the Reiki energy.

So are you ready to find out the difference that Reiki can make to your life?

Disclaimer

Introduction

By using this book, you accept this disclaimer in full.

No advice

The book contains information. The information is not advice and should not be treated as such.

No representations or warranties

To the maximum extent permitted by applicable law and subject to section below, we exclude all representations, warranties, undertakings and guarantees relating to the book.

Without prejudice to the generality of the foregoing paragraph, we do not represent, warrant, undertake or guarantee:

- that the information in the book is correct, accurate, complete or non-misleading.

- that the use of the guidance in the book will lead to any particular outcome or result.

Limitations and exclusions of liability

The limitations and exclusions of liability set out in this section and elsewhere in this disclaimer: are subject to section 6 below; and govern all liabilities arising under the disclaimer or in relation to the book, including liabilities arising in contract, in tort (including negligence) and for breach of statutory duty.

We will not be liable to you in respect of any losses arising out of any event or events beyond our reasonable control.

We will not be liable to you in respect of any business losses, including without limitation loss of or damage to profits, income, revenue, use, production, anticipated savings, business, contracts, commercial opportunities or goodwill.

We will not be liable to you in respect of any loss or corruption of any data, database or software.

We will not be liable to you in respect of any special, indirect or consequential loss or damage.

Exceptions

Nothing in this disclaimer shall: limit or exclude our liability for death or personal injury resulting from negligence; limit or exclude our liability for fraud or fraudulent misrepresentation; limit any of our liabilities in any way that is not permitted under applicable law; or exclude any of our liabilities that may not be excluded under applicable law.

Severability

If a section of this disclaimer is determined by any court or other competent authority to be unlawful and/or unenforceable, the other sections of this disclaimer continue in effect.

If any unlawful and/or unenforceable section would be lawful or enforceable if part of it were deleted, that part will be deemed to be deleted, and the rest of the section will continue in effect.

Law and jurisdiction

This disclaimer will be governed by and construed in accordance with Swiss law, and any disputes relating to this disclaimer will be subject to the exclusive jurisdiction of the courts of Switzerland.